Dengue Hemorrhagic Fever

Vaccine for Dengue Fever

Johanne E. Phillips

Table of Contents

Hemorrhagic dengue

In medicine, DHF is Dengue Hemorrhagic Fever.

It's a fever caused by the Dengue virus by Aedes mosquitos and it mostly affects children under 10 or 15 years

Dengue fever hemorrhagic, also known as severe dengue, is a potentially life-threatening condition that can develop as a complication of dengue fever. In this article, we will explore the causes, treatment options, and preventive measures for dengue fever hemorrhagic, shedding light on the imjpportance of understanding and addressing this severe manifestation of the disease.

Dengue fever is a viral illness caused by the dengue virus, which is transmitted to humans through the bites of infected mosquitoes, primarily the Aedes aegypti mosquito. This disease can affect people of all ages and can have varying degrees of severity.

Dengue fever is primarily found in tropical and subtropical regions, where the climate favors the breeding of mosquitoes. The dengue virus has four distinct serotypes and infection with one serotype provides lifelong immunity to that specific serotype but only temporary immunity to the other three. This means that individuals can experience dengue fever multiple times in their lifetime.

Causes of Dengue Fever Hemorrhagic:

Dengue fever hemorrhagic is caused by infection with the dengue virus, specifically transmitted through mosquito bites, primarily by the Aedes mosquito species. There are four distinct serotypes of the dengue virus, and contracting one type does not provide immunity against the others. Secondary infections with a different serotype can increase the risk of developing dengue fever hemorrhagic. The abnormal immune response to the virus triggers inflammation and damage to blood vessels, leading to bleeding and the severe symptoms associated with dengue fever hemorrhagic.

Brazil Dengue fever

Dengue fever has surged in Brazil's hot rainy season, forcing health authorities to take emergency measures and start mass vaccination against the mosquito-borne illness.

In the first five weeks of this year 364,855 cases of infection have been reported, the Health Ministry said, four times more than dengue cases in the same period of 2023.

The rapid spread of dengue has caused 40 confirmed deaths, the ministry said, and a further 265 are being investigated.

Brazil has bought 5.2 million doses of the dengue vaccine Qdenga developed by Japanese drugmaker Takeda's (4502.T),with another 1.32 million doses provided at no cost to the government, a ministry statement said.

Three Brazilian states have declared emergencies, including the second most populous state Minas Gerais, and the Federal District, where the capital Brasilia is located and is facing an unprecedented rise in infections.

Brasilia will start vaccinating children aged 10-14 on Friday with Qdenga, the local government said on Wednesday.

Cases of dengue in Brasilia since the start of the year have exceeded the total for the whole of 2023, with a rate of infection of 1,625 cases per 100,000 inhabitants, compared to the national average of just 170.

Army troops have been deployed in the capital to help track breeding spots of the Aedes aegypti mosquito that carries and spreads the dengue virus in homes and backyards wherever there is stagnant water.

The Brazilian Air Force set up a field hospital in preparation for a surge in cases needing hospital care in Ceilandia, a densely-populated poor suburb of Brasilia.

Cities such as Rio de Janeiro that are preparing to celebrate Carnival starting on

Saturday have taken measures to prevent an epidemic.

The Health Ministry has set up an emergency center to coordinate operations against dengue across Brazil.

World Health Organization (WHO) director-general Tedros Adhanom, said this dengue outbreak has been fueled by the El Niño phenomenon that brought increased rainfall in Brazil.

"This current dengue outbreak is part of a large global increase in dengue fever with over 500 million cases and over 5,000 deaths reported last year from 80 countries in every region of the world except Europe," he said at a ministry event.

South America is seeing a surge in cases of dengue during the southern hemisphere summer, exacerbated by rising temperatures and the El Nino weather pattern in the Pacific that contribute to prolonged dengue seasons and spread of infections, scientists say.

Dengue fever symptoms include a high fever, headache, vomiting, muscle and joint pains, and an itching skin rash. In some cases, the disease can cause a more severe hemorrhagic fever, resulting in bleeding that can lead to death.

Causes of Dengue hemorrhagic fever

Dengue fever is caused by any one of four types of dengue viruses. You can't get dengue fever from being around an infected person. Instead, dengue fever is spread through mosquito bites.

The two types of mosquitoes that most often spread the dengue viruses are common both in and around human lodgings. When a mosquito bites a person infected with a dengue virus, the virus enters the mosquito. Then, when the infected mosquito bites another person, the virus enters that person's bloodstream and causes an infection.

After you've recovered from dengue fever, you have long-term immunity to the type of virus that infected you — but not to the other three dengue fever virus types. This means you can be infected again in the future by one of the other three virus types.

Your risk of developing severe dengue fever increases if you get dengue fever a second, third, or fourth time.

Dengue (DENG-gey) fever is a mosquito-borne illness that occurs in tropical and subtropical areas of the world. Mild dengue fever causes a high fever and flu-like symptoms. The severe form of dengue fever, also called dengue hemorrhagic fever, can cause serious bleeding, a sudden drop in blood pressure (shock), and death.

Millions of cases of dengue infection occur worldwide each year. Dengue fever is most common in Southeast Asia, the western Pacific islands, Latin America and Africa. But the disease has been spreading to new areas, including local outbreaks in Europe and southern parts of the United States.

Researchers are working on dengue fever vaccines. For now, in areas where dengue fever is common, the best ways to prevent infection are to avoid being bitten by mosquitoes and to take steps to reduce the mosquito population.

Dengue hemorrhagic fever symptoms

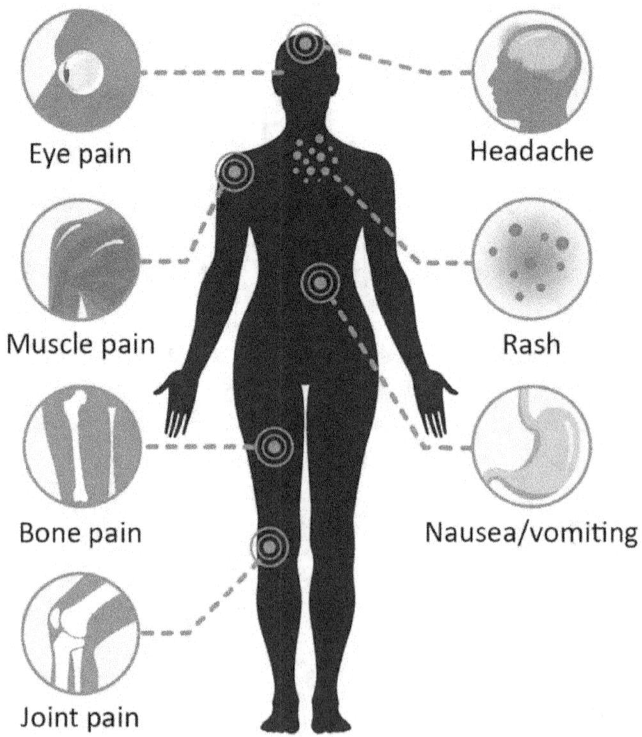

1. **Headache and Eye Pain:** One of the initial symptoms of dengue fever is a severe headache, often accompanied by pain behind the eyes. This symptom can be persistent and worsen with movement.

2. **High Fever:** Dengue fever is characterized by a sudden high fever, typically exceeding 101°F (38.5°C). The fever may last for several days and is often accompanied by chills and sweating.

3. **Severe Joint and Muscle Pain:** Dengue fever is also known as "breakbone fever" due to the intense joint and muscle pain it causes. This pain can be debilitating and make even simple movements difficult.

4. **Nausea and Vomiting**: Many dengue fever patients experience nausea, vomiting, and loss of appetite. These gastrointestinal symptoms can contribute to dehydration and weakness.

5. **Skin Rash:** A rash may develop on the skin, usually two to five days after the onset of fever. It typically appears as small red

spots or patches and may be accompanied by itching.

6. **Fatigue and Weakness**: Dengue fever often leaves patients feeling fatigued and weak, even after the fever subsides. This can persist for several weeks, affecting the individual's ability to carry out daily activities.

Severe Symptoms and Complications

In some cases, dengue fever can progress to severe forms, including Dengue Hemorrhagic Fever (DHF) and Dengue Shock Syndrome (DSS). These conditions require immediate medical attention and can be life-threatening if left untreated.

Dengue Hemorrhagic Fever is characterized by bleeding, blood plasma leakage, and low platelet count. Symptoms may include severe abdominal pain, persistent vomiting, bleeding from the nose or gums, blood in urine or stool, and difficulty breathing.

Dengue Shock Syndrome involves a sudden drop in blood pressure, leading to shock. Symptoms include intense abdominal pain, disorientation, cold and clammy skin, weak pulse, and a rapid drop in urine output.

Vaccine for dengue fever

After a person is infected with dengue, they develop an immune response to that dengue subtype. The immune response produces specific antibodies to that subtype-specific surface proteins that prevent the virus from binding to macrophage cells (the target cells that dengue viruses infect) and gaining entry. However, if another subtype of dengue virus infects the individual, the virus will activate the immune system to attack it as if it were the first subtype. The immune system is tricked because the four subtypes have very similar surface antigens. The antibodies bind to the surface proteins but do not inactivate the virus. The immune response attracts numerous macrophages, which the virus proceeds to infect because it has not been inactivated. This situation is referred to as Antibody-Dependent Enhancement (ADE) of a viral infection. This makes the viral infection much more acute. The body releases cytokines that cause the endothelial tissue to become permeable which results in Dengue Haemorrhagic Fever (DHF) and fluid loss from the blood vessels.

There are several possibilities to explain the phenomenon:

1. A viral surface protein laced with antibodies against a virus of one serotype binds to a similar virus with a different serotype. The binding is meant to neutralize the virus surface protein from attaching to the cell, but the antibody bound to virus also binds to the receptor of the cell, the Fc-region antibody receptor FcγR. This brings the virus into proximity to the virus-specific receptor, and the cell endocytoses the virus through the normal infection route.

2. A virus surface protein may be attached to antibodies of a different serotype, activating the classical pathway of the complement system. The complement cascade system

instead binds C1q attached to the virus surface protein via the antibodies, which in turn bind the C1q receptor found on cells, bringing the virus and the cell close enough for a specific virus receptor to bind the virus, beginning infection. This mechanism has not been shown specifically for the dengue virus infection but is supposed to occur with Ebola virus infection in vitro.

3. When an antibody to a virus is present for a different serotype, it is unable to neutralize the virus, which is then ingested into the cell as a sub-neutralized virus particle. These viruses are phagocytosed as antigen-antibody complexes, and degraded by macrophages. Upon ingestion, the antibodies no longer even sub-neutralize the body due to the denaturing condition at the step for acidification of phagosome before fusion with the lysosome. The virus becomes active and begins its proliferation within the cell.

In 1997, 205 cases of DHF/DSS occurred in Cuba, all in people older than 15 years, after an infection with DENV-2 serotype. All but three cases were shown to have been previously infected by the DENV-1 virus, during the epidemic of 1977–1979. Two outbreaks of the disease occurred after the first epidemic in 1977-1979, one in 1981 and one in 1997. People who had been infected with DENV-1 during the 1977-79 outbreak and secondarily infected with DENV-2 in 1997 had 3 to 4 more chances to develop a severe disease than those secondarily infected with DENV-2 in 1981. While heterotypic antibody titers decrease, homotypic antibody titers increase during long periods (4 to 20 years). This could be due to the preferential survival of long-lived B memory cells producing homotypic antibodies, thanks to their bigger affinity. This cross-reactive protection does not persist for more than 3 months. The decrease of cross-reactive neutralizing antibody titers in the serum could be the reason for more severe secondarily infections.

There are currently several vaccines available for the prevention of dengue fever, a viral illness transmitted by mosquitoes. The effectiveness of these vaccines can vary depending on the specific vaccine and the individual being vaccinated.

One vaccine, called Dengvaxia, was developed by Sanofi Pasteur and was the first vaccine to be licensed for the prevention of dengue fever. This vaccine is effective in preventing dengue fever in individuals who have previously been infected with the virus. However, it is not as effective in individuals who have not previously been infected.

Another vaccine, called TAK-003, was developed by Takeda and is effective in preventing dengue fever in individuals who have previously been infected with the virus.

It has also been shown to be effective in preventing severe dengue fever in individuals who have not previously been infected.

Both of these vaccines are designed to protect against all four types (or serotypes) of the dengue virus. It is important to note that no vaccine is 100% effective and that individuals who have been vaccinated may still be at risk of getting dengue fever.

It is important to talk to a healthcare provider about the benefits and risks of dengue fever vaccination and to consider factors such as the likelihood of exposure to the virus, the potential severity of the disease, and individual risk factors.

Dengue hemorrhagic fever prevention

Treatment for Dengue Fever Hemorrhagic: Effective treatment of dengue fever hemorrhagic requires prompt medical intervention. Hospitalization plays a vital role, allowing healthcare professionals to closely monitor the patient's condition. Regular assessments of vital signs, blood counts, and organ function help detect any changes or complications associated with dengue fever hemorrhagic. By providing timely medical care, interventions can be initiated to manage the condition effectively.

One key aspect of treatment is fluid replacement therapy. Dengue fever hemorrhagic can cause significant fluid loss, leading to dehydration and electrolyte imbalances. Intravenous fluid administration is crucial for restoring and maintaining proper hydration levels in patients. Blood transfusions may also be necessary in cases of severe bleeding or low platelet counts. The aim is to replenish blood components and support the body's ability to clot effectively.

In addition to fluid management, symptomatic relief is important for managing dengue fever hemorrhagic. Pain relievers, such as acetaminophen, can help reduce fever and alleviate body aches. However, it is important to avoid nonsteroidal anti-inflammatory drugs (NSAIDs) and aspirin, as they can increase the risk of bleeding complications. Close monitoring of the patient's condition is essential to detect any signs of organ dysfunction or worsening bleeding.

Prevention of Dengue Fever Hemorrhagic:

Preventing dengue fever is crucial in reducing the risk of developing dengue fever hemorrhagic. Implementing preventive measures, such as eliminating mosquito breeding sites, using mosquito repellents, wearing protective clothing, and employing mosquito control strategies like insecticide-treated bed nets, are vital in preventing mosquito bites and subsequent dengue virus infection. By focusing on community-wide efforts to raise awareness and practice proper hygiene, we can collectively reduce the incidence of dengue fever and its severe complications, including dengue fever hemorrhagic.

Mosquito Repellent

Mosquito repellents, when used as directed, are generally considered safe for humans. The active ingredients in most mosquito repellents are designed to deter mosquitoes and other insects, reducing the risk of mosquito-borne illnesses such as malaria, Zika virus, dengue fever, and West Nile virus.

Common active ingredients in mosquito repellents include DEET (N, N-diethyl-meta-toluamide), picaridin, IR3535, and oil of lemon eucalyptus. These ingredients have been extensively studied for safety, and when used according to the product instructions, they are generally regarded as safe for most people, including pregnant women and children.

However, it's essential to follow these guidelines when using mosquito repellents:

Read and Follow Instructions: Always read and follow the instructions on the product label. Pay attention to the recommended application frequency and any age restrictions.

Appropriate Application: Apply the repellent to exposed skin or clothing, as directed. Avoid applying it to cuts, wounds, or irritated skin.

Avoiding Eyes and Mouth: Take care to avoid applying repellent near the eyes, mouth, and on the hands of young children.

Use in Well-Ventilated Areas: When using aerosol or spray repellents, do so in well-ventilated areas to minimize inhalation.

Wash Off After Use: When you return indoors, wash treated skin with soap and water.

Choose Appropriate Concentrations: Consider the concentration of the active ingredient in the repellent. Higher concentrations generally provide longer protection, but it's important to choose a concentration suitable for the situation.

While mosquito repellents are generally safe, some individuals may experience skin irritation or allergic reactions. If you have concerns or if irritation occurs, discontinue use and consult a healthcare professional.

It's worth noting that there are alternative methods to reduce mosquito exposure, such as wearing long sleeves and pants, using mosquito nets, and avoiding outdoor activities during peak mosquito activity times. If you have specific health concerns or conditions, it's advisable to consult with a healthcare professional for personalized advice.

Conclusion:

Dengue fever hemorrhagic is a severe manifestation of dengue fever that necessitates immediate medical attention. By understanding the causes, prompt diagnosis, and appropriate treatment options, healthcare professionals can effectively manage dengue fever hemorrhagic and mitigate its potentially life-threatening complications. Furthermore, emphasizing preventive measures such as mosquito control and community education is essential in reducing the incidence of dengue fever and its associated complications. Through collaborative efforts, we can work towards minimizing the impact of dengue fever hemorrhagic and protecting the health and well-being of individuals and communities.

Japan's Takeda in regulatory talks to launch dengue

BENGALURU (Reuters) -Japan's Takeda Pharmaceutical is holding talks with Indian regulators to make its dengue vaccine available in the country, the drugmaker's global head of vaccines, Gary Dubin, told Reuters on Tuesday.

"We are in talks with regulators and plan to start a clinical trial very soon," said Dubin.

The Japanese drugmaker plans to scale up the production of its dengue vaccine Qdenga through a partnership with Indian vaccine maker Biological E., the companies said earlier in the day.

These vaccines will be available for governments in endemic countries by 2030 as part of their national immunization programs.

"One of the challenges we have is being able to scale up manufacturing to support what we expect will be a very large global need," Dubin told Reuters, adding that the collaboration is aimed at doubling Takeda's current capacity to manufacture the vaccine.

Biological E. will ramp up its capacity to produce 50 million doses a year, accelerating Takeda's efforts to produce 100 million doses per year within the decade, the companies said.

Dubin said Biological E has the technical expertise to manufacture the vaccine.

Takeda's dengue vaccine is available for children and adults in countries like Indonesia, Thailand, Argentina, and Brazil, but is not approved for use in India.

Brazil has bought 5.2 million doses of Qdenga, with an additional 1.32 million doses provided at no cost, as the country undertakes emergency measures and mass vaccinations against the mosquito-borne disease.

Since the beginning of 2023, the world has been facing an upsurge in dengue cases and deaths reported in endemic areas, with further spread to areas previously free of dengue, according to the World Health Organization.

The Global Health Agency estimates more than five million dengue cases and over 5,000 associated deaths have been recorded across all six WHO regions.